MELATONIN
THE MIRACLE FOR LIFE

Terry Lemerond
Foreword by Jacob Teitelbaum, M.D.

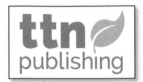

ttn
publishing

Library of Congress Cataloging-in-Publication Data is on file with the Library of Congress.

ISBN: 978-1-952507-05-2

Design: Gary A. Rosenberg • www.thebookcouple.com
Editor: Kathleen Barnes • www.takechargebooks.com

Printed in the United States of America

10   9   8   7   6   5   4   3   2   1

Contents

Foreword

Greetings! I'm Jacob Teitelbaum, M.D., an integrative physician, a board-certified specialist in internal medicine with deep interest in chronic fatigue syndrome, fibromyalgia, sleep and chronic pain. I battled chronic fatigue and fibromyalgia myself during my stressful years in medical school in the '70s, so I'm very familiar with the destructive effects these conditions have on body, mind and spirit. In my struggle to find healing for myself, I also discovered my life's passion: for those who already have serious health conditions, to help them find natural healing, and improved quality of life and vibrant well-being. Best of all, I hope I can help others prevent the debilitating illnesses so many others have suffered by offering them wise lifestyle choices.

If you're a seeker of natural ways of health and healing, you may already be familiar with Terry Lemerond. I consider him to be the "Oprah" of Natural Health, being the first to see what is coming over the horizon and making it available to the public.

I've had the distinct pleasure of knowing and working with Terry for more than 20 years. I have the deepest respect for his expertise, particularly his knowledge of supplements, herbs and all of the pharmacopeia of healing plants and molecules that our modern world has forgotten. In its quest for synthetic answers to age-old health problems and new challenges, modern medicine has lost is way. It has failed to understand the synergy between nature and the human body.

Thankfully, Terry Lemerond is the catalyst to bring us back to our roots, quite literally. That's why I've teamed with him on this book, to bring melatonin out of the shadows of just being for sleep when in fact, it can have profound benefits for our entire body. Melatonin is critical not only as an antioxidant, but for setting our day-night cycles. This book will inform you about the far-reaching and impressive healing effects of melatonin, which Terry will share with you in his inimitable style. You'll find that this book contains a unique section in which I collaborated with Terry to advise readers to share with their physicians of melatonin's impressive healing powers.

So now is the time to wake up to the impressive and largely disregarded health benefits of melatonin. Welcome to this exciting journey!

—Jacob Teitelbaum, M.D.
Kailua-Kona, Hawaii

CHAPTER 1

Meet Melatonin—
It's for More Than Just ZZZs

Most of us know about melatonin. Or at least we think we do. "Melatonin? Isn't that to help you sleep?" you might ask. Very few of us know anything more about this nutrient that offers profound beneficial effects to the entire human organism.

Yes, melatonin does help you sleep. A good night's rest is essential to many areas of general health, including blood sugar control, weight control and yes, immune function.

But melatonin's health benefits go much farther than simply promoting a good night's rest for a wide variety of reasons.

Researchers have long known the link between melatonin and a host of health benefits, especially in older people, but for some unexplained reason, our attention has been rivetted on the sleep aspect of melatonin and we've ignored unique and substantial scientific evidence that melatonin does more, so much more.

Primary among melatonin's wonders is immune system enhancement. In Chapter 2, you'll learn all about strengthening your immune system with melatonin as well as the large body of scientific evidence that supports its use as an antiviral and antimicrobial in today's challenging world.

Melatonin also has an uncanny ability to help turn back the clock on the aging process. The process is not yet well understood, but the effects have been documented. We'll give you the big picture in Chapter 3.

All of this information is immensely exciting. In all my years of researching the benefits of a broad range of nutrients, I haven't seen such convincing scientific evidence of broad beneficial effects with virtually no serious side effects.

I'll go out on a limb and say that because of melatonin's broad effects to the benefit of nearly all systems and cells in the human body, almost everyone should take melatonin, especially those over 50.

What exactly is melatonin?

Melatonin has been called a hormone, and indeed it does have hormone-like properties as a chemical messenger. Technically known as N-acetyl-5-methoxytryptamine, melatonin acts like a hormone in every way except that it can actually be extracted from food. It is mainly produced by the pineal gland, a pea-sized gland in the center of the brain. True hormones are only manufactured by the human body. More about that in a few paragraphs.

But, Dr. Walter Pierpaoli, one of the world's foremost anti-aging researchers, insists melatonin is not a true hormone. He's the first to admit, as a decades-long melatonin researcher, that we don't know exactly what melatonin is, but we do know what it does.

Dr. Pierpaoli calls melatonin the "master mediator of all hormones" and the "universal chemical mediator of the biological world." He even enthusiastically calls it "the miracle molecule." It's also been called the "molecular handyman," meaning it can do just about everything. All of that is pretty impressive! But does melatonin live up to all the hype? In a single word, "Yes."

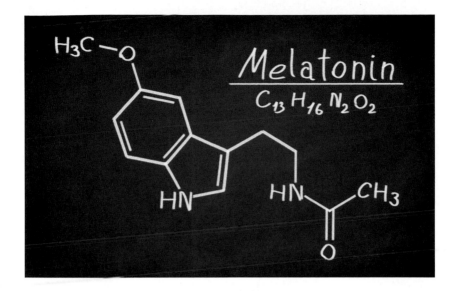

Among the things we do know:

❖ Like hormones, melatonin is produced in many parts of the body.

❖ It is connected to circadian rhythms, the day-night/sleep-wake cycle, produced by the pineal gland in darkness.

❖ It is the messenger of the pineal gland, the body's "aging clock" to send a message of youth throughout the body, preventing the devastating degeneration we know as aging, Dr. Pierpaoli says.

❖ It can also be produced by the gut and the retina of the eye.

❖ It is absorbed through the digestive system from a wide variety of foods, including many fruits, vegetables, grains, nuts, seeds, eggs and fish. No hormone is absorbed through food, which is one of the reasons why melatonin cannot be accurately described as a hormone.

❖ Melatonin levels reach their peak at puberty and diminish as we age.

❖ It helps break the physiological stress cycle that can result in a plethora of degenerative diseases associated with aging.

Over the past few decades, there has been an abundance of top-quality research on melatonin. In fact, nearly 28,000 studies have been published on melatonin, more than on any natural product. Yet somehow, the value of melatonin as a sleep aid has overshadowed its other enormously impressive benefits. Somehow it has flown under the radar of public awareness. Now it's time to change that.

What else melatonin can do

In addition to turning back the clock on aging, here's a brief list of the scientifically proven effects of melatonin supplements. We'll go into them in detail in the coming chapters.

Antiviral: Melatonin has been confirmed as a virus fighter, even against the potent SARS and MERS viruses. It has been shown to strengthen immune function to prevent all type of infections and to reduce the severity of the infection if you get one, whether it's viral, bacterial, or even parasitic. Melatonin is especially helpful in strengthening the immune systems of older people who are more vulnerable to infections.

Heart health: Studies show that melatonin reduces artery clogging cholesterol levels, helps keep blood pressure at normal levels and counteracts harmful heart-damaging stress hormones called corticosteroids.

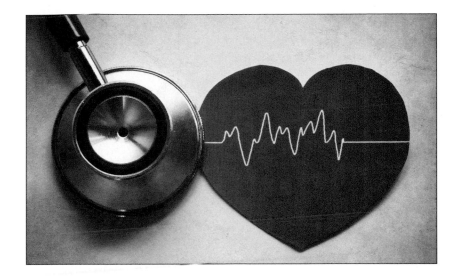

Cancer prevention: Immune system boosting T-cells are the body's primary cancer fighters. By preventing or slowing the decline of the immune system as we age, melatonin protects your body from cancer by improving the body's ability to identify and eradicate cells that might turn cancerous. There is also research that shows melatonin is particularly effective in preventing hormonally-related cancers, including breast and prostate cancer. For those who have cancer, melatonin should not be taken during chemotherapy, but taken before and after chemotherapy. Melatonin may help protect bone marrow cells from the destructive effects of chemo.

Researchers from Baylor University also found that melatonin overcomes cancer patients' almost inevitable resistance to 5-fluorouracil, a chemotherapy drug often used to treat colorectal and other cancers.

Sexual health: The anti-inflammatory and anti-oxidative stress effects of melatonin have been shown to help reverse erectile dysfunction in men. It also increases the probability of success for in vitro fertilization treatments and increases the chance of survival for embryos when both men and women are undergoing hormonal enhancement treatment.

Control type 2 diabetes: It's shown to improve insulin uptake and blood sugar control, especially in older people. It has also been shown to improve the effectiveness of oral anti-diabetes medication as well as preventing some of the more terrible side effects of diabetes, including heart disease and blindness.

Eye health: Melatonin has been researched and found effective in treating and preventing a variety of eye diseases, including macular degeneration and glaucoma.

Gastrointestinal health: The GI tract produces 400 times as much melatonin as the pineal gland. Among its powerful effects is giving relief to sufferers from Irritable Bowel Syndrome (IBS) and Inflammatory Bowel Disease (IBD).

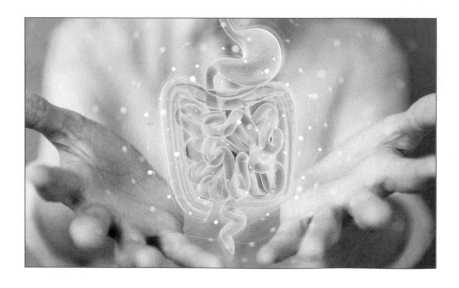

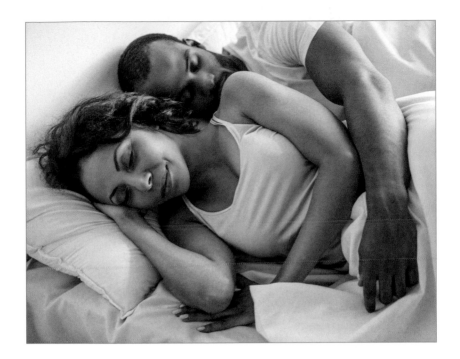

Treat fibromyalgia and chronic fatigue syndrome: Studies show melatonin relieved chronic pain in sufferers of both of these disorders and improved quality of life because of better sleep.

Treat infections: Clinical data shows that melatonin successfully treats sepsis, a potentially fatal infection in newborns, and herpes viral infections.

Sleep disorders, of course: These include insomnia, non 24 sleep/wake disorder, jet lag and sleep disorders caused by pharmaceuticals used for other conditions, including blood pressure. This is partly because it helps restore circadian rhythm, the body's natural sleep cycle.

WHAT YOU NEED TO KNOW

Melatonin is most commonly used quite effectively for sleep disorders, especially insomnia, but it is little known for its considerable other health-enhancing effects, including:

☑ Increasing levels of Natural Killer (NK) cells and T-cells, specialized white blood cells that are at the forefront of infection fighting. Melatonin has been clinically proven to increase the immune system's ability to fight off viral, bacterial, microbial and parasitic infections.

☑ Some of the same immune system boosting cells also make melatonin a powerful weapon against cancer, especially breast and prostate cancer.

☑ Melatonin has also been shown in human studies to be effective in preventing and treating:

☑ Heart disease

☑ Type 2 diabetes

☑ Eye diseases like macular degeneration and glaucoma

☑ Digestive problems including Irritable Bowel Syndrome and Inflammatory Bowel Disease

☑ Fibromyalgia and chronic fatigue syndrome

☑ Infections, including the herpes virus and sepsis in newborns

CHAPTER 2

Today's Important Melatonin Message

Let's take a few paragraphs here to delve a bit more deeply into the relationship of melatonin and the immune system and what it means in today's infectious disease environment.

Melatonin is a bit of a scientific mystery. As you'll remember from Chapter 1, it acts like a hormone, a chemical messenger, but it does not fulfill the technical definition because melatonin can be obtained through food sources.

Among the things we do know about melatonin is that the human body manufactures it in darkness. This is part of the reason it is helpful as a sleep aid and to help people suffering from jet lag. The manufacture of melatonin in the dark is one of the reasons to have your bedroom as dark as possible and to keep television and other light-emitting devices out of your bedroom.

So, we need to be able to naturally make melatonin, get some from food sources and sometimes we need a boost, especially when we are at risk of various viral infections. That's a good reason to take a melatonin supplement. More about that later.

Acclaimed melatonin researcher Russel J. Reiter, Ph.D., of the University of Texas Health Science Center in San Antonio, as far back as 1996 wrote in his book, *Melatonin: Breakthrough Discoveries That Can Help You,* "...melatonin is a dominant player in the immune system. The discovery is only a few years old, but researchers are already demonstrating melatonin's ability to treat cancer, slow the progression of AIDS, make the body more resistant to colds, and protect the immune system from the toxic effects of chemotherapy."

Now we know that melatonin is a potent antiviral. As far back as 2013, Italian researchers urged the scientific community to conduct further research on melatonin's potential as a virus fighter.

The immune system is immensely complex. Part of its makeup is an alphabet soup of specialized white blood cells called lymphocytes designed to attack "invaders." These invaders are usually pathogens, like viral, bacterial, parasitic or other microbial infections.

Among these are NK or Natural Killer cells. Don't you love that term when we're talking about knocking out possibly deadly infections? NK cells are specialized white blood cells that are the immune system's first line of defense against viral infections and cancer cells.

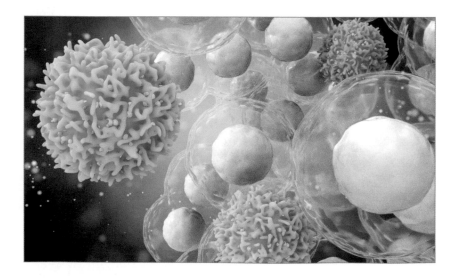

Other immune cells called T-cells are produced by the thymus gland. They not only help build a strong immune system, they provide the immune system's power punch to eliminate the infection or the growth of tumor cells. Highly effective T-cells wipe out the infections that the NK cells have flushed out and made vulnerable. Active and healthy T-cells are essential for survival. With the decline in our number of T-cells as we age, we need something to help us shore up the defenses.

Melatonin is part of the answer, that's for sure.

Melatonin plays a key role in enhancing both of these types of disease-fighting cells. Key 2006 research from a consortium of scientists from around the world confirmed melatonin's role in enhancing the immune system, and says it "has the potential to be useful" in enhancing immune system function and preventing cancerous tumor formation.

As we age, our immune systems weaken. That's why common infections like the flu and pneumonia tend to be worse and even more deadly in older people. Aging immune systems sometimes have difficulty differentiating between "good" pathogens, including bacteria, viruses and more importantly, the "bad" ones.

It's interesting that white blood cells, the first line of defense in the immune system, have melatonin receptors, although scientists aren't exactly sure why. We do know that natural levels of melatonin produced by the pineal gland, the gut and the retina of the eye diminish as we age. We also know that melatonin helps stimulate the release of cytokines, small proteins that help attack infections and reduce inflammation. We also know that people with the highest blood levels of melatonin are far more able to fight off serious infections.

Finally, and perhaps most importantly in today's world, melatonin is a potent antiviral, shown to knock out a wide variety

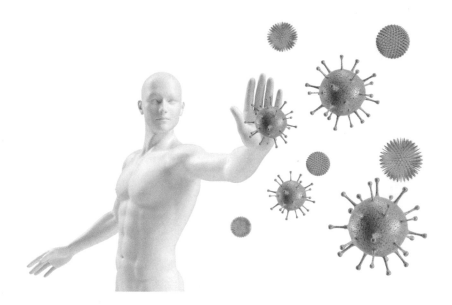

of deadly viral diseases, including SARS, MERS, avian flu and more. New research strongly suggests melatonin may be a power-ful, natural weapon against the most serious viruses without side effects.

Inflammation and oxidative stress

Inflammation is the body's natural response to an irritant. It could be a splinter in your finger that turns red and sore or a twisted ankle that swells up and feels hot. Or, it could be a response to a germ or a virus that your immune system perceives as a foreign invader.

Oxidative stress is your body's response to the presence of free radical oxygen molecules that create an imbalance in your body's ecosystem and open it to a high risk of disease. Among the many downstream effects of oxidative stress is damaged DNA and imperfect reproduction of cells, leading to disease like cancer, type 2 diabetes, heart disease, rheumatoid arthritis and more.

Melatonin's healing powers are surely connected to its well-researched anti-inflammatory and antioxidant properties, but there is most likely something else at work here.

Researchers theorize that melatonin's success in combating viruses may be connected to reining in the immune system's overreaction to viruses and the inflammation that frequently accompanies them, leading to deadly pneumonias, respiratory failure and sometimes death. Researchers have long been confounded by reasons for the gradual deterioration of the immune system as we age.

As far back as 2005, a multi-national team of researchers concluded that melatonin is a key part of healthy immune function in the elderly and immunocompromised people, those most likely to become the most ill from viruses.

An article published in the journal *Life Sciences* in June 2020 was among the most exciting research on melatonin and the immune system. A consortium of American and Chinese researchers (including Dr. Reiter) concluded, "There is significant data showing that melatonin limits virus-related diseases."

In an article in *Frontiers in Medicine* in May of 2020, Dr. Reiter wrote, "Melatonin's multiple actions as an anti-inflammatory, antioxidant, and antiviral (against other viruses) make it a reasonable choice for use. Melatonin is readily available, can be easily synthesized in large quantities, is inexpensive, has a very high safety profile and can be easily self-administered."

Another study, published in May of 2020 suggested that melatonin might also reduce the severity of symptoms of deadly viral diseases.

Andrographis and melatonin

So, let's talk for a moment about adding melatonin to andrographis, an Ayurvedic herb with its own impressive immune boosting powers. The idea is right on track with a consortium of American scientists who asked the same question and came up with a hopeful answer as early as August of 2020 in a study published in the journal *Life Sciences.*

They concluded, "Considering the properties of both compounds in terms of anti-inflammatory, antioxidant, antipyrogenic, antiviral and ER stress modulation and computational approaches revealing andrographolide docks with the SARS-CoV2 binding site, we predict that this combination therapy may have potential utility against (even the most deadly viruses)."

Sorting out the scientific lingo for a moment here, they think the combination of andrographis and melatonin could work together to prevent and treat the most deadly viruses that challenge all of us today. As of this writing, we are still early in the pandemic research game, but this is an exciting development that has the potential to save many lives.

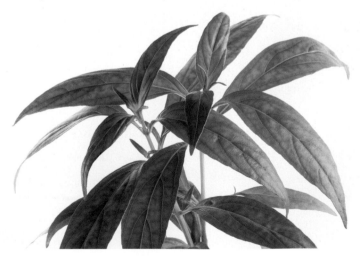

WHAT YOU NEED TO KNOW

Melatonin is a well-researched, immune system enhancer:

☑ It increases the body's production of Natural Killer (NK) cells and T cells, the foundational molecules of the immune system.

☑ It is anti-inflammatory and an antioxidant, enhancing its effectiveness against all kinds of infections, including viral infections.

☑ Early research suggests that melatonin can safely reduce the number of viral infections, including COVID-19 infections, especially in elderly people whose immune systems have degraded with age.

☑ A combination of melatonin and the Ayurvedic herb, andrographis, may prove to be a potent treatment for the pandemic virus.

CHAPTER 3

Melatonin for Long Life

Sometimes called, the "time-keeping hormone," I might more accurately call melatonin the "Merlin" hormone after the Medieval wizard whose aging clock ran backwards. Wouldn't that be nice?

Think of the human aging process as a clock that slooooowly winds down over time. But what if melatonin keeps that clock strongly ticking along regardless of age?

Scientists have long known that aging is closely linked with the human body's circadian rhythms, the human brain's internal day-night clock. But circadian rhythms are much more than just sleeping at night and being awake in the daylight.

As we know from Chapter 1, melatonin is a quasi-hormone that directs a wide range of body functions. It certainly stands to reason that a healthy immune system would translate to a longer life, but melatonin gives us more than that.

In humans, circadian rhythms coordinate mental and physical systems throughout the body, says the National Sleep Foundation. "The digestive system produces proteins to match the typical timing of meals and the endocrine system regulates hormones to suit normal energy expenditure."

The iconic study of melatonin and longevity came all the way back in 1985 when Dr. Pierpaoli and his colleague Georges Maestroni discovered that simply adding a tiny amount of melatonin

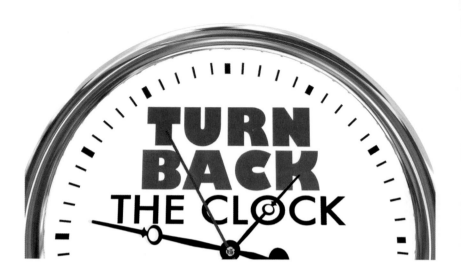

to the drinking water of tiny shrews living in their lab extended their lives by an amazing 20 percent! Their brethren showed typical signs of aging. They became frail and lifeless, losing hair and disengaged from life, but the melatonin shrews were strong and glossy almost until the end.

So if that could be translated to human years, it would add more than 15 years to the average lifespan of an American. What if you could be nearly assured of 94 years instead of 78 years? What would you do with those 15 years, especially if you were otherwise very healthy?

Why do we age?

There are numerous theories why we age:

1. Cell damage over time

2. Gradual deterioration of the immune system

3. Breakdown of the body's internal timing mechanisms

You've probably already figured this out: Melatonin addresses all three.

So while there are multiple paths to aging and eventual death, melatonin's trifold strengths are the perfect combination for a long and healthy life.

Antioxidant properties: By wiping out free radical oxygen molecules, the underlying cause of many of the most serious diseases of aging, melatonin may actually prevent or at least lessen the severity of Alzheimer's disease, various types of cancer, Parkinson's disease, heart disease and crippling arthritis.

Immune system stimulation: We've already talked about melatonin's immune enhancing abilities in Chapter 2. There is no doubt that melatonin protects us from invasion by pathogens, but also balances the immune system when it overreacts and causes autoimmune diseases.

Restoration of circadian rhythms: We've mentioned this before, but it bears repeating that the balanced day-night cycle had a profound effect on your entire body. As Dr. Reiter says, "Once our biological rhythms falter, the body can no longer function in an efficient manner. We're like antique sports cars badly in need of a tune up, prone to breaking down by the side of the road."

Anti-inflammatory: Inflammation is a fourth element that is critical to the aging process. It is an underlying cause of many, if not most, of the diseases of aging, including heart disease, type 2 diabetes, Alzheimer's disease and most types of cancer. Melatonin is unquestionably a potent anti-inflammatory, an important bonus to its trifecta against aging.

Then there are those mitochondria...

Mitochondria, the body's tiny furnaces that supply energy to every single cell, are key to the aging process, as you might well imagine. While they are technically called organelles, mitochondria perform a very specific function within a cell. Dr. Reiter's research published in 2018 (yes, he's been pursuing melatonin for more than 25 years!) confirms that the mitochondria not only have higher concentration of melatonin than other organelles, but that mitochondria actually produce melatonin.

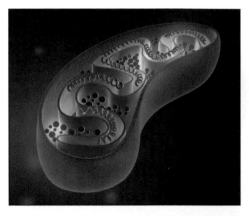

Research shows that the mitochondria in our cells produce melatonin

To translate the scientific gobbledygook: Melatonin is concentrated in the body's most elementary energy producing system, wiping out free radical oxygen molecules with a direct effect on the aging process.

Dr. Reiter concluded in that study: "Thus, melatonin is optimally positioned to scavenge the radicals and reduce the degree of oxidative damage. In light of the 'free radical theory of aging,' including all of its iterations, high melatonin levels in mitochondria would be expected to protect against age-related organismal decline. Also, there are many age-associated diseases that have, as a contributing factor, free radical damage. These multiple diseases may likely be deferred in their onset or progression if mitochondrial levels of melatonin can be maintained into advanced age."

Gender preference

And it seems that women have a bit of an advantage over men when it comes to melatonin and the benefits it brings. We know that melatonin levels drop in women when they reach menopause, but more recent research suggests that older women still have more natural melatonin production than older men. Dr. Reiter theorizes this may account, at least in part, for women's longer life expectations.

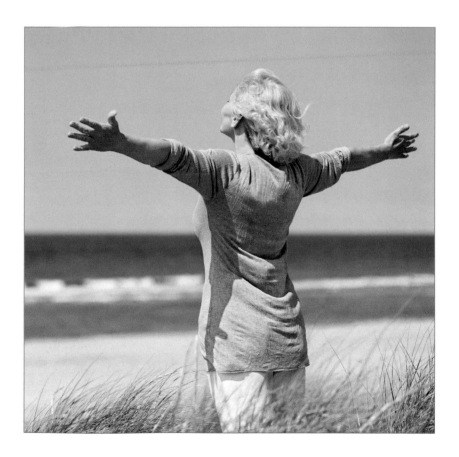

Stay Young by Maintaining a Healthy Circadian Rhythm

While we don't have full control over our circadian rhythm, here are some healthy sleep tips to improve your 24-hour sleep cycles.

Seek out sun: Exposure to natural light, especially early in the day, helps reinforce the strongest circadian cue.

Follow a consistent sleep schedule: Varying your bedtime or morning wake-up time can hinder your body's ability to adjust to a stable circadian rhythm.

Get daily exercise: Activity during the day, preferably outside, can support your internal clock and help make it easier to fall asleep at night.

Avoid caffeine: Stimulants like caffeine keep you awake and throw off the natural balance between sleep and wakefulness. Everyone is different, but if you're having trouble sleeping, you should avoid caffeine after 12:00 noon.

Limit light before bed: Artificial light exposure at night can interfere with circadian rhythm. Experts advise dimming the lights and putting down electronic devices in the hour before bedtime.

Keep naps short and early in the afternoon: Late and long naps can push back your bedtime and throw your sleep schedule off-kilter.

These steps to improve sleep hygiene can be an important part of supporting a healthy circadian rhythm, but other steps may be necessary depending on the situation. If you have persistent or severe sleeping problems, daytime drowsiness, and/or a problematic sleep schedule, it's important to talk with a doctor who can best diagnose the cause and offer the most appropriate treatment.

WHAT YOU NEED TO KNOW

Melatonin is well known for its anti-aging properties because:

☑ As an antioxidant, it destroys free racial oxygen molecules, the underlying cause of many diseases of aging including heart disease, cancer, diabetes and Alzheimer's disease.

☑ It enhances immune function, leaving the whole human organism stronger and more able to resist a wide range of infection, including potentially fatal viral and bacterial pneumonias.

☑ It supports a healthy circadian rhythm, keeping body mechanisms in life-sustaining balance.

☑ It is a powerful anti-inflammatory, combating the underlying inflammation that is another underlying cause of most of the diseases of aging.

AND

☑ It strengthens the mitochondria, the body's cellular energy furnaces, keep your cells young and healthy.

CHAPTER 4

Melatonin
and a Healthy Heart

Heart disease is the most common disease in the Western world and the #1 killer in the United States.

Most of us know someone with high blood pressure, high cholesterol, irregular heart rhythms, clotting and clogging of the arteries, or even someone who has had a heart attack or stroke. Maybe you have experienced some of these health challenges yourself. If so, you have a place among the 30.3 million Americans or about 12% of the population with some form of heart disease.

It's serious. Heart disease is the cause of one in four deaths in America. It can strike any time, almost without notice. It claims 647,000 lives a year, almost half of them from sudden death. I admit, those are daunting statistics.

It is true that numerous pharmaceutical and natural ways of addressing heart disease have increased life expectancy in people with heart disease. Traditional medicine and modern science have identified numerous ways to extend the lives of those diagnosed with a wide range of cardiovascular diseases.

So where does melatonin fit into this picture?

Circadian rhythms

Let's start with your body clock, the day-night pattern that governs vital body functions. You'll remember from Chapter 1 that the pineal gland produces melatonin *and* controls circadian rhythms. Melatonin is deeply connected to the biological clock that governs the endocrine gland system, the chemical messenger system that governs virtually every body process.

The sleep-wake cycle is the most familiar of the circadian rhythms, but the biological clock also governs the regulation of body temperature and a whole array of hormonal functions including blood sugar metabolism, eating habits, fertility, digestion and much more.

Out-of-balance circadian rhythms have been linked to obesity, diabetes, sleep disorders, depression, bipolar disorder and seasonal affective disorder, which can, in turn, spawn a host of other serious health issues.

It turns out that melatonin is at the heart of a solution for all of the above, including heart function.

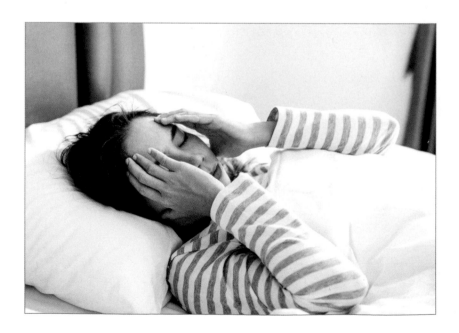

Melatonin's unique ability to regulate circadian rhythms is a big part of the answer, but there are other factors in play here. Since Dr. Reiter's book in 1996, a large body of research has confirmed that melatonin promotes heart health in a variety of ways:

Lowers blood pressure: It turns out that there is even a circadian rhythm to blood pressure, which can be as much as 20% lower at night than in the daytime. The connection of melatonin to that lower overnight blood pressure is well established and science now confirms that high melatonin levels actually are protective against those early morning heart attacks. The anti-inflammatory and blood vessel relaxing effects of melatonin are also credited with helping people with high blood pressure return their numbers to normal.

In one of Dr. Reiter's animal studies, animals with high blood pressure that were given melatonin had their levels drop by an impressive 21%. A Polish study on people with metabolic syndrome (that deadly triple whammy of abdominal fat, high blood pressure, high cholesterol and elevated blood sugar) who took just 5 mg of melatonin before bed for two months lowered their systolic blood pressure (the upper number) by an average of 12.3 points and diastolic (bottom number) by 6.5 points.

Lower cholesterol and triglycerides: When your blood fats are too high, they clog arteries. The buildup of fat in arteries, called arteriosclerosis, can partly or totally block arteries, potentially leading to a heart attack, stroke or heart failure.

In a nutshell, a substantial body of research shows that melatonin supplementation reduces dangerous blood fats, including low density lipoprotein (LDL) cholesterol and triglyceride blood fats. It has also been proven to increase HDL (good cholesterol), making melatonin a powerful tool against disease causing metabolic syndrome.

More about this in coming chapters, but melatonin's ability to help control weight is also a factor in lowering cholesterol and lowering the risk of heart disease.

In an analysis of a vast array of studies published in the journal *Clinical Nutrition* in 2018, the authors drew the firm conclusion, "Melatonin supplementation has significant effects on triglycerides and total cholesterol levels, which was more evident in higher dose and longer duration . . ."

Another study published in *Clinical Nutrition* in 2019, confirmed melatonin's positive effects on HDL cholesterol, and perhaps more importantly, confirmed that in people with diabetes who are at high risk of heart disease, it is effective in reducing many conditions known to contribute to heart disease.

Clotting and clogging: Here's a pretty amazing factoid about the human body, compliments of Dr. Reiter: The bone marrow produces blood platelets that can clump together and act as "Band-aids" in case of an injury, rushing to the site of an injury and closing off injured blood vessels to prevent excessive bleeding. However, platelets can become too sticky and clump together in your arteries (atherosclerosis) and cause an obstruction. Alternatively, sometimes the platelets "decide" to become slippery to prevent clumping. Then there is a danger of excessive bleeding. So . . . the body, in its wisdom, "decides" that the body is less likely to be injured at night, so the platelets are more slippery, thereby opening arteries and preventing heart attacks and strokes. Then, as the sun rises and the likelihood of injury increases, platelets become more sticky to prevent excessive bleeding if there is an injury. So what does melatonin have to do with all of this? Scientists believe that melatonin

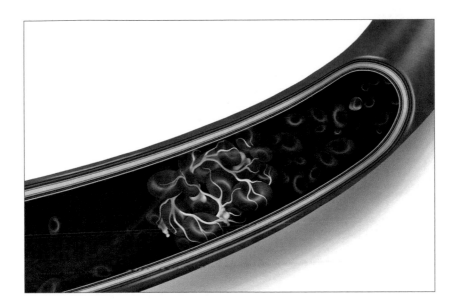

is responsible for the slippery vs slick night-day transformation. In fact, a 1991 study found that blood platelets immersed in a melatonin solution reduced their clumping by 85%.

Isn't nature fascinating?

In short, melatonin has been well-researched for its anti-clotting action. In fact, if you are already taking blood thinners, you should consult with your doctor before starting to use melatonin because it could be necessary to adjust or even completely eliminate your blood thinner dosage, but don't do it without medical advice.

Heart rhythms: Arrhythmias, irregular, afib (atrial fibrillation) are all risk factors for heart attack, stroke, heart failure and other heart problems.

Melatonin's sleep normalizing properties are part of melatonin's positive effect on heart rhythms. We know that people who are sleep deprived are more likely to have heart rhythm irregularities, so it stands to reason that better sleep means better heart rhythms. But it is more than that.

It's also known that irregular heart rhythms are less common at night, a direct effect of melatonin like we see with all of the other heart-related issues.

Heart attacks and strokes: Melatonin is an antioxidant, capable of profound protection against free radical oxygen molecules that are a major underlying cause of the diseases of aging, including heart disease. During a heart attack, the heart muscle is deprived of critical blood flow and oxygen. This results in tissue damage and a flood of free radicals, causing further damage and potentially causing strokes. Melatonin's free radical scavenging powers can limit the damage and the possibility of another heart attack or stroke.

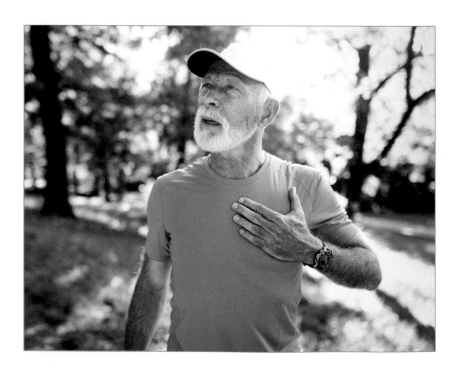

An interesting aside: It has long been known that very few heart attacks happen at night, when melatonin levels are highest. (Remember that melatonin is produced by the pineal gland in complete darkness.) There is a "heart attack zone" between 6 a.m. and noon, peaking at 9 a.m., the times when melatonin levels are the lowest.

It's a great example of the circadian rhythm. At night, typically you are lying down and sleeping and your pulse and breathing slow, blood pressure drops and even cholesterol declines. But as soon as the sun comes up, your body "clock" signals it is time to get ready for an active day, your heart rate increases, blood pressure and cholesterol rise.

Way back in 1996, Dr. Russel Reiter wrote in his book, *Melatonin: Breakthrough Discoveries That Can Help You*, "Melatonin appears, in fact, to have a direct protective effect on the heart and circulatory system in general. What's more, there is growing evidence that declining levels of melatonin—both the abrupt fall that occurs in the morning and the gradual overall decline that accompanies aging—are hazardous to the heart."

Here's another fascinating factoid: Doctors have noticed that heart attack patients who are hospitalized in an ICU have slower recoveries. Yes, indeed, these patients have no doubt had more serious heart damage, but it raises an obvious question to students of melatonin: If the patients were not in the ICU's bright light 24 hours a day and their bodies were able to naturally produce more melatonin, might they recover faster?

WHAT YOU NEED TO KNOW

Melatonin is a well-researched heart protective hormone-like molecule.

Science shows that melatonin:

- ☑ Lowers blood pressure

- ☑ Lowers "bad" cholesterol

- ☑ Raises "good" cholesterol

- ☑ Lowers blood fat levels

- ☑ Reduces blood clotting that can block arteries and cause heart attacks and strokes

- ☑ Restores irregular heart rhythms

CHAPTER 5

Melatonin Against Cancer

Cancer is a terrible disease that modern medicine has yet to conquer.

Despite billions upon billions of dollars spent on research, billions spent on health care and an untold toll in human lives, the cure eludes us.

Current wisdom suggests that every cancer is bio-individual. That's scientific language for everyone is different and all cancers are different and, therefore, effective cancer treatment can take a wide range of paths.

Yet, of course, there are some common threads.

All cancers:

❖ Are the result of the failure of the system that governs the natural life spans and reproduction of all cells, a process called apoptosis;

❖ Create a network of blood vessels to sustain and nourish cancerous cells, a process called angiogenesis;

❖ Spread to other body systems, a process called metastasis.

The disease with many faces

Most of us know someone who has cancer and, sadly, many of us know someone who has died of cancer.

The National Cancer Institute reports that 1,762,450 new cases of cancer were diagnosed in 2019 and 606,880 people died of the disease.

The most common types of cancer in the U.S. are (in descending order, according to estimated new cases in 2019):

❖ breast

❖ lung and bronchial

❖ prostate

❖ colorectal

❖ melanoma

❖ bladder

❖ non-Hodgkin's lymphoma

❖ kidney and renal

❖ endometrial

❖ leukemia

❖ pancreatic

❖ thyroid

❖ liver

Where does melatonin fit in this picture?

At the risk of minimizing the already impressive benefits of melatonin detailed in the previous four chapters, I'll dare say that the "Master Hormone's" preventive and healing properties are at their peak when it comes to cancer.

Science is discovering more and more that the most effective, cancer-fighting nutrients are those that target the disease from multiple directions.

Melatonin certainly fits that bill.

But let's step back for a moment and take a look at cancer itself and how it kills.

Cancer is an interruption in the natural process of cell life and death. All cells are born and die. On average, all of the cells in your body are replaced every seven to 10 years. You are quite literally born again! Colon cells turn over every four days, while the cells in your skin are completely replaced every 28 days, muscle cells every 15 years and heart muscle cells every 40 years. Other cells, like brain cells, can actually survive 200 years, longer than any of us will live.

So why do we age? One of the reasons we age is that cells reproduce themselves imperfectly. They do not always create perfect copies of themselves. Those imperfect reproductions, over time, become parents of new cells that are less perfect and so on.

Apoptosis: For reasons science does not totally understand, old cells do not die on schedule and live beyond their natural lifespans. Colon cells live beyond their pre-programmed four-day lifespan, skin cells beyond 28 days and so on. Through this process, called apoptosis, old cells literally keep growing and creating more and more new cells, some of which may be cancerous. These

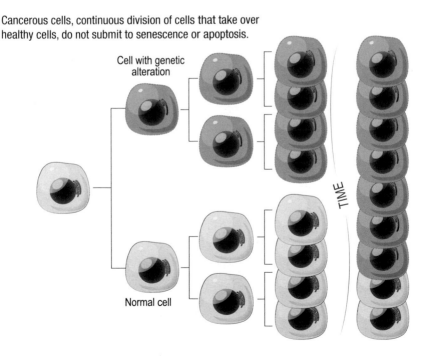

Cancerous cells, continuous division of cells that take over healthy cells, do not submit to senescence or apoptosis.

cancerous cells crowd out new healthy cells and begin to affect body functions.

While cancers grow differently and at different speeds in different parts of the body, the beginning process is always the same: uncontrolled cellular growth.

So, what if there was a way to re-establish normal cell growth, cell division and cell death? Or to prevent apoptosis from starting cancerous cellular growth at all?

You've probably already guessed that melatonin fits that bill and brings with it many more weapons in the anticancer arsenal.

Italian research confirms that melatonin promotes apoptosis and, because of its antioxidant properties, counteracts the toxicity of chemotherapy agents. This means it increases the effectiveness of chemotherapy, even in patients with advanced lung, breast, gastrointestinal, and head and neck cancers. It also reduced the long term and serious side effects of chemotherapy drugs, including heart problems, nerve damage, anemia, profound fatigue and more.

While research on the underlying reasons why melatonin is effective against cancer in many ways, there seems to be agreement that its antioxidant and anti-inflammatory powers play an important role in cancer prevention and treatment.

Here are a few ways cancer takes hold and spreads and how melatonin addresses the problem:

Angiogenesis: Like all living things, cancerous tumors need nutrients. They get these nutrients by creating their own network of blood vessels that feed the tumor and help it grow, a process called angiogenesis.

Melatonin restricts the tumors' ability to feed themselves by cutting off the blood vessel network.

Normal cells   Cancer cells

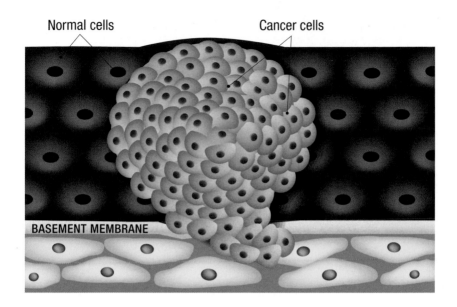

BASEMENT MEMBRANE

A 2019 pivotal Chinese study says melatonin may be an important anticancer agent because it cuts off the blood to that network, thereby eradicating the tumor's nutrient supply. This seems to be particularly effective against solid tumors like those found in breast and lung cancers, the most deadly cancers in the Western world.

An Iranian study in 2017 also found that melatonin enhances the ability of chemotherapy agents to stop that blood vessel growth.

Metastasis: Most of us have heard this term. It is simply the spread of cancer from one part of the body to another. For example, breast cancer often spreads to the lungs, liver and bones. Lung cancer most typically spreads to the adrenal glands, bones and brain. Most cancers will metastasize if they are not stopped before they can spread. That is why it is so important to stop cancer at the stages of apoptosis and angiogenesis. But once cancer has spread, it is not the end.

Metastasis: How Cancer Spreads

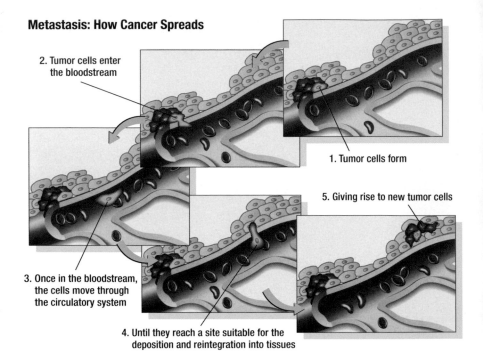

2. Tumor cells enter the bloodstream

1. Tumor cells form

5. Giving rise to new tumor cells

3. Once in the bloodstream, the cells move through the circulatory system

4. Until they reach a site suitable for the deposition and reintegration into tissues

Melatonin has well-documented anti-metastatic properties. Dr. Reiter's 2017 study not only confirms that melatonin prevents metastasis, it works synergistically with conventional agents against the most deadly cancers.

Epigenetics: Epigenetics are a fairly recent discovery that is somewhat complex. I won't bog you down with too much information, so here it is in a nutshell: We know that genetics, the traits we were born with, determine everything from the color of our eyes to our risk for a wide variety of diseases. Epigenetics are the outside influences that we all encounter in our everyday lives that can have many negative effects, including turning off the genes that naturally suppress cancer. These epigenetic factors can be everything from air pollution to what's in our drinking water. They are also governed by our personal choices in food, our home environments, and in the case of melatonin, nighttime lighting.

We all know by now that melatonin is produced by the pineal gland in complete darkness. But in the modern world, artificial lighting, television lighting and our various devices emit light late into the hours of darkness when we should be producing melatonin.

That blockage of melatonin production seems to be an epigenetic trigger for the formation of a variety of types of cancerous tumors. Fortunately, research tells us that this epigenetic problem is reversible by increasing available melatonin. This could take place through extended time spent in complete darkness and/or through supplements.

In conclusion

"There is highly credible evidence that melatonin mitigates cancer at the initiation, progression and metastasis phases," wrote a consortium of University of Texas, Spanish, Mexican and Taiwanese researchers. "What is rather perplexing, however, is the large number of processes by which melatonin reportedly restrains cancer development and growth. These diverse actions suggest that what is being observed are merely epiphenomena (secondary effects) of an underlying, more fundamental action of melatonin that remains to be disclosed."

The scientific lingo for the concept that melatonin is a powerful anticancer agent and researchers don't really know why. Not yet, anyway. Stay tuned.

WHAT YOU NEED TO KNOW

Extensive scientific evidence confirms that melatonin:

☑ Stops the wild cell division that causes cancerous tumors

☑ Stops the formation of blood vessels that feed cancerous tumors

☑ Stops the spread of cancer

☑ Reverses genetic damage caused by lifestyle choices that slow the body's ability to make melatonin

☑ Enhances the effectiveness of conventional chemotherapy drugs

CHAPTER 6

Melatonin for Sexual Health and Much More

Remember those circadian rhythms that govern the night/day, sleep/wake cycles?

Well, now I'm going to blow your mind and tell you that there are season rhythms that have profound effects on the human body and many of them on sexual health and fertility.

Backing up just a bit, you'll remember that melatonin is produced by the pineal gland in darkness, bringing on restorative sleep. (Sleep—I know. We're coming to that in the next chapter.)

So think about this: Perhaps the lengths of the day and night have something to do with human reproduction?

We already know this is so in animals. Animals that hibernate or go into semi-hibernation in the winter time really are not sexually active during that period. Think about this: Long winter nights and high melatonin production = less ovulation. Dr. Reiter even mentions that Inuit women, who live in Alaska and northern Canada where there is no daylight in winter, even stop their menstrual cycles in winter when melatonin levels are very high. In fact, most mammals become sexually active—and fertile—in the spring. It is a logical process. Adults may starve in the winter, but by spring, there is more food, and by summer, when the young are born, there is usually abundant food, improving the survival rate of their young. On the reverse side of that coin, there was a time about 20 years ago when farmers sometimes used melatonin to delay ovulation in their livestock so the young would be born on the farmer's timetable.

Could this be true for humans, too? It is possible, even though there isn't much research to prove it. The jury is still out in many cases, but Dr. Reiter has weighed in on the side of melatonin. In a 2013 study, he concluded, "In general, the direct actions of melatonin on the gonads and adnexa (adjacent organs) of mammals indicate it is an important agent for maintaining optimal reproductive physiology."

Here's what we do know:

A remedy for PMS? Premenstrual syndrome and its uncomfortable symptoms, including bloating, headache, fatigue and mood swings, is the scourge of women of childbearing age. A 2012 study from Douglas Mental Health University in Montreal confirmed that women with the worst form of PMS, called Premenstrual Dysphoric Disorder (PMDD) had low nighttime melatonin levels.

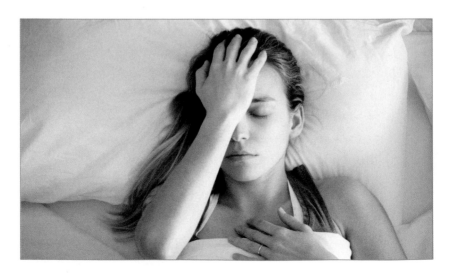

A treatment for unexplained infertility: In 2019, Spanish scientists determined that moderate doses of melatonin given to women who could not conceive for unknown reasons were slightly more likely to have successful in vitro fertilizations and live births when they were given either 3 mg or 6 mg of melatonin supplements daily.

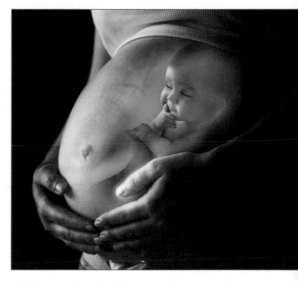

Australian research suggests that melatonin may be part of a successful treatment plan for infertility. Egyptian researchers confirmed that men with fertility problems also had low melatonin levels, suggesting that melatonin supplementation might improve their chances of conception.

Treat erectile dysfunction? Men with erectile dysfunction (ED) have been known to have low melatonin levels, so it stands to reason that increased amounts of melatonin may remedy the problem. It is known that, contrary to popular belief, most erectile dysfunction has underlying physical causes, not psychological ones. A 2018 Turkish study of men with mild, moderate and severe ED suggests that further study of melatonin to diagnose and treat ED would be valuable, and a Chinese study the same year went a little farther and suggested that melatonin's antioxidant powers might help overcome neuropathy and sexual dysfunction in men with type 2 diabetes.

Raise or lower sperm count? There are conflicting studies about whether melatonin improves or decreases sperm count. One study suggests that melatonin added to sperm increased the likelihood of fertilization of an egg during in vitro fertilization.

Contraceptive? Melatonin was even briefly used in an estrogen-free human contraceptive over 20 years ago, but results were too variable for it to be reliable, so the idea was abandoned.

You will note that the above studies are fairly vague. There is much research still to be done on melatonin and sexual health in both men and women.

There's much more...

Here's a brief synopsis on the many other diseases and conditions for which melatonin has been used and scientifically validated.

Prevent or delay age-related macular degeneration: A pivotal 2005 study published in the *Annals of the New York Academy of Sciences* confirmed that elderly patients who took supplements with just 3 mg of melatonin daily had healthier retinas and delayed the onset of macular degeneration, a common cause of blindness in the elderly, without negative side effects.

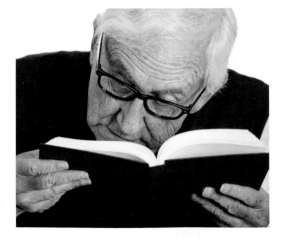

Migraine prevention: An exciting article published in the *Journal of Family Practice* recommended that doctors encourage their patients with chronic migraines to take 3 mg of melatonin every night. Melatonin has been shown to be at least as effective in migraine prevention as amitriptyline (Elavil) with their headache days

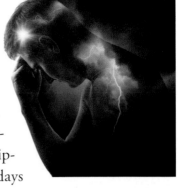

per month reduced by 50% or more. Best of all, the headache reduction came without side effects, unlike other medications used for migraines.

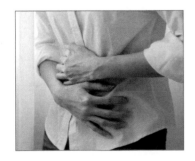

Relieve heartburn and stomach ulcers: At least three studies confirm melatonin offers relief from the pain of ulcers and heartburn, especially when used along with omeprazole (Prilosec), a common over-the-counter treatment for heartburn.

Autism: Canadian researchers found that melatonin helped people on the autism spectrum cope better with life. Yes, the researchers confirmed, improved sleep quality was part of the effect, but for unknown reasons, helped people with Autism Spectrum Disorder with other side effects of their condition: anxiety,

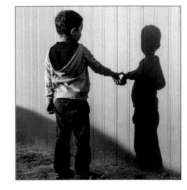

pain, depression, and gastrointestinal disorders.

Aid with the withdrawal from benzodiazepines: Benzodiazepines (Valium, Zanax, Klonopin), used to treat insomnia, anxiety, seizures, bipolar disorder and schizophrenia, are among the most

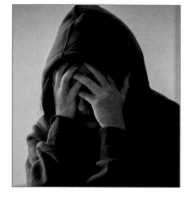

addictive pharmaceuticals known. Withdrawal from the addiction is terribly painful. Danish research published in 2016 confirms the value of melatonin in helping people addicted to "benzos," even those with severe mental illnesses, to withdraw slowly and without associated insomnia and other side effects.

Reduce ear ringing: Also known as tinnitus, this annoying condition often robs its victims of sleep. Researchers at Ohio State University confirmed that men with tinnitus who took 3 mg of melatonin before bed for just 30 days experienced significant reduction in the level of tinnitus and better sleep quality.

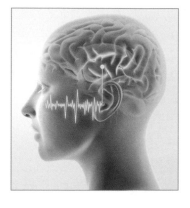

I believe what we know about melatonin and its amazing capabilities will expand dramatically in the coming years. Right now, there are more than 33,000 scientific published studies on melatonin. Hundreds, perhaps thousands, more will increase our knowledge and understanding of this hormone-like natural substance and how and why it works. This is just the tip of the iceberg of what may inarguably become the most important nutritional supplement of our times.

WHAT YOU NEED TO KNOW

The research on melatonin is extensive and surprising. Among the things we know:

☑ It increases fertility in both men and women and can improve the chances of a live birth from in vitro fertilization.

☑ It relieves symptoms of PMS and even the much more debilitating PMDD.

☑ It can reduce erectile dysfunction.

And we should all watch for additional scientific confirmation of these impressive effects:

☑ Prevent and treat macular degeneration.

☑ Migraine prevention.

☑ Relief from heartburn and gastric ulcers.

☑ Treatment of symptoms of autism.

☑ Aid in withdrawal from benzodiazepines.

☑ Reduce or even eliminate tinnitus.

CHAPTER 7

And Melatonin for Sleep, of Course!

Most people think of melatonin as a sleep aid. We've learned in this book that this "handyman molecule" does so much more. Yet that iconic reputation for sleep enhancement is well deserved.

The Centers for Disease Control and Prevention (CDC) says that at least one-third of Americans get less than the recommended seven hours of sleep a night. Seven in ten of us confess to lacking sufficient sleep at least once a month and 11% report they never get enough sleep. Lack of restorative sleep leads to short-term problems like daytime drowsiness, distraction, impaired memory, loss of productivity and a greater risk of automobile accidents.

Sure, missing out on a few hours of shuteye occasionally isn't a big deal. You can generally make it up with an early bedtime for a couple of nights. But when that occasional lack of sleep becomes habitual, it leads to serious, long-term health problems including obesity, depression, diabetes, immune system compromise, heart attack and stroke.

If you suffer from occasional or chronic sleeplessness, you know there are two different types of insomnia. First, there is the type when you have difficulty falling asleep, and second is the type where you fall asleep without a problem, but then find yourself wide awake four or five hours later.

What keeps us awake

Why are we staying awake at night? Stress is probably the number 1 reason for sleeplessness. How many times have you awakened at 3 a.m. thinking about that report you have due at work or financial challenges or your kid's poor grade on a test, or these days, the risks of serious illness? Sure, there are other reasons for insomnia, including too much light in your room (so your body can't naturally produce melatonin), screen time close to bedtime, a room that is too warm or too cold, the effects of some medications, choices in the use of caffeine and alcohol, a bad mattress and much more. There are answers to all of those problems.

Conventional medicine offers some dangerous pharmaceutical remedies. Sleeping pills like Ambien, Sonata, Halcion, Restoril, Lunesta are virtually all addictive and have serious side effects

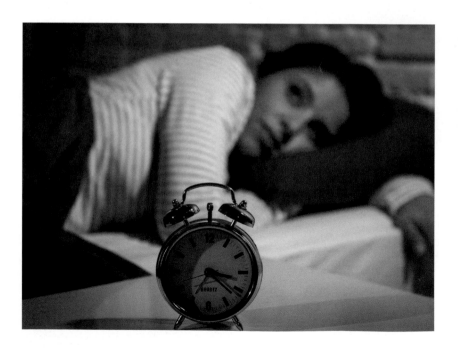

including driving and eating while asleep, severe and sometimes life-threatening allergic reactions, memory loss, daytime drowsiness and more.

Antidepressants are frequently used to treat insomnia as well, with equally dire side effects. Primary among them are highly addictive benzodiazepines (Elavil, Sinequan, Desyrel). Their side effects include thoughts of suicide, irregular heartbeat, memory loss, severe headaches and weight gain.

It's not a pretty picture, is it? So what can you do if you find yourself counting sheep night after night?

Since you're reading this book, you already know: Take melatonin, a natural hormone-like molecule that is well-documented as a reliable sleep aid with no serious side effects.

How melatonin works

Melatonin gently brings your body into sleep mode and helps it stay that way, especially if you use a time release form.

It works by easing your body into the appropriate circadian rhythm. That's one of the reasons why it is so helpful for overcoming jet lag and helping your body adjust to a new time zone. This is also why melatonin helps shift workers who must sleep in the daytime.

Melatonin begins to be produced by your body when it gets dark, giving a signal to your body that it is time to sleep. It also binds to brain chemicals to help reduce nerve activity. It also reduces levels of the brain chemical dopamine that keeps you awake. We also know that the pineal gland's production of melatonin decreases with age, explaining why many older people have sleep problems.

Here's a synopsis of what extensive research shows:

❖ An important Brazilian meta-analysis (review of high-quality published studies) confirmed melatonin's three-fold benefits in sleep disorders: decreasing the amount of time it took to fall asleep, increasing total sleep time and increasing sleep quality.

❖ Australian researchers joined many others in confirming the value of melatonin supplementation in helping promote sleep on time and helping subjects stay asleep. It's interesting that many studies used a very low dosage—5 mg—and found significant, positive results.

❖ We already know from Chapter 6 that melatonin actually helps patients withdraw from the highly addictive benzodiazepines that are often used to treat insomnia and, in reality, worsen the problem.

❖ A consortium of researchers from Britain, the U.S. and Israel documented that melatonin was effective and safe for children on the autism spectrum, who frequently have sleep disorders. The 2017 study showed melatonin shaved nearly 40 minutes from the time it took them to fall asleep and helped them stay asleep nearly an hour longer.

❖ Plentiful research confirms that melatonin helps people with a wide variety of health challenges, including strokes, traumatic brain injuries, and heart attacks improve their sleep quality.

Other ways to make sure you get a good night's sleep

There are lots of ways to improve your sleep time and sleep quality, all of which will go hand-in-hand with melatonin supplementation.

Sometimes called sleep hygiene, these simple actions are essential tools to beat insomnia:

Consistency: Going to bed at approximately the same time and having the same wake-up time every day gets your circadian rhythms into balance and improves sleep quality.

Wind down before bedtime: Take a half hour or so to wind down, turn down the lights, maybe put on some soft music, meditate or even take a warm bath. All of these will start your natural melatonin production.

Stay away from blue screens for an hour before bedtime: That means stop using tablets, phones and gaming devices at least an hour before sleep time. Some devices (like Kindles) have blue screen blockers, so they're fine for bedtime reading. TV is OK if you are at least six feet away from the screen. (An aside here: Plan your nighttime reading and device use well. Thrillers, high speed games and even the news may not be your best choices.)

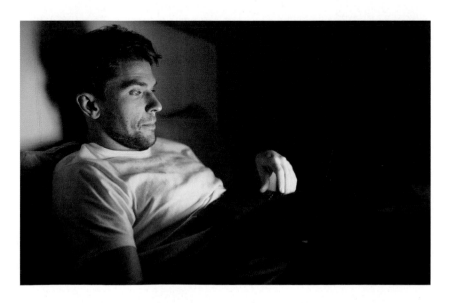

Darken your room: Making your bedroom as dark as possible will also stimulate melatonin production. If there are streetlights or neighbor's lights outside your window, consider room-darkening shades. Even nightlights can disturb your natural melatonin production. A tip for those who make nighttime bathroom visits: Keep a flashlight beside your bed instead of having nightlights on all the time.

Cut the sound, too: As much as possible, block sound from other rooms in your home, traffic outside, neighbor noise, etc. You may need ear plugs or a white noise machine.

Avoid caffeine after 2 p.m.: You will probably know your tolerances. Some people find that any caffeine after noon will disrupt their sleep. Caffeine isn't just in coffee. It's in tea and in many soft drinks.

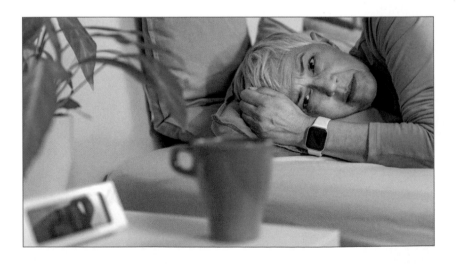

Reduce alcohol consumption: Alcohol may help you fall asleep, but it disrupts sleep patterns and can cause you to awaken at the wrong time.

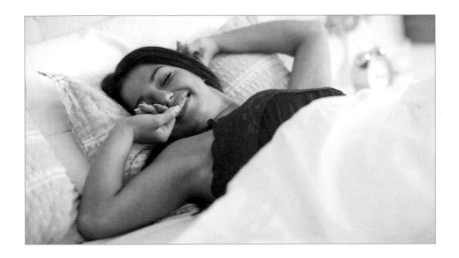

Don't eat too late: You should finish eating at least two hours before bedtime, preferably longer. If you lie down too soon after eating, you risk heartburn. Also, your digestive system gets revved up trying to handle a meal, which can interfere with sleep.

Be physically active, but not right before bedtime: For your overall health, please be physically active, but exercise too close to bedtime causes your heart rate to rise and sends your body into wake-up mode. However, a little bit of gentle yoga stretching can also relax you and put you into sleepy time mode.

Get outside in the daytime: Exposure to sunlight will help keep those circadian rhythms on track.

Turn down the thermostat: Keeping your bedroom cool improves sleep quality.

Avoid tossing and turning: If you find yourself lying awake in the middle of the night for more than 10 minutes, get up, listen to some soothing music, meditate, or drink a cup of non-caffeinated herbal tea (chamomile is excellent to relax you).

WHAT YOU NEED TO KNOW

Melatonin is an effective, safe and scientifically validated sleep aid.

It has been confirmed to:

- ☑ Decrease the time it takes to fall asleep
- ☑ Help you stay asleep all night
- ☑ Improve sleep quality

Poor sleep causes a host of serious health problems, including:

- ☑ Obesity
- ☑ Diabetes
- ☑ Heart Disease
- ☑ Depression

It's especially effective in people with:

- ☑ Autism
- ☑ Traumatic brain injuries
- ☑ Strokes
- ☑ Heart attacks

CHAPTER 8

Know How to Make the Right Choice

Some people swear by melatonin's almost mystical ability to help them get restorative sleep while others are adamant that melatonin has no effect on their ability to sleep. Still others say they don't need it because they have no trouble sleeping. In any case, when you look at the overwhelming body of evidence presented in this book, you'll see that the benefits of melatonin go far beyond helping you sleep.

In fact, I'll go out on a limb and say that almost everyone will benefit from melatonin's hormone-like activities, its ability to re-establish circadian rhythms and its anti-inflammatory, immune-enhancing effect, whether or not you have any trouble sleeping. It's worth taking melatonin supplements.

It will probably make you sleepy

That's a good thing at night but not such a good thing in the daytime when you may need to drive, work, take care of kids or conduct other business. Please be aware that any melatonin supplement you take will work with your body's natural melatonin production and will probably cause you to feel sleepy, so please use it correctly. That means taking melatonin an hour or two before you plan to go to bed and not during the day when you need to be alert.

Melatonin has a half-life of 40–60 min, meaning half of it is eliminated from your body within 40 to 60 minutes, half of the remaining amount in another hour and so on. Since most of us want to sleep for 7 to 8 hours, which is why it's a good idea to find a product that is labelled "sustained release." These types of melatonin will be particularly helpful 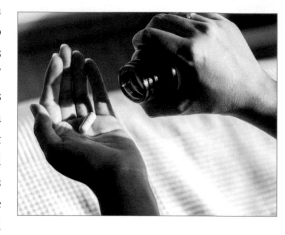 for people who wake up in the middle of the night and have trouble getting back to sleep.

The melatonin I use every night is 10 mg of a very active, sustained-release ingredient called EP120. I do believe that everyone should take melatonin nightly, whether or not they sleep well. Melatonin is required in every metabolic function of our bodies. It is the keep-well and stay-well molecule that prevents and treats multiple health conditions.

Melatonin strength: What should I take?

The strength of melatonin you decide to take is really an individual choice based on your own unique needs.

For Basic Immune Support

I recommend a 10mg sustained-release tablet each night to reestablish your circadian rhythms, bolster your immune responses and moderate psychological well-being.

For extra support, especially for extra strong immune defense, reduction of tumor and cancer risk and recovery from periods of sleep deprivation like travel of hectic schedules, I believe that a 20 mg melatonin is best.

After all, there have been numerous clinical studies that show higher daily amounts are extremely safe and beneficial. Based on nearly 27,000 studies, the consensus is that melatonin is safe, non-toxic and a required molecule needed by all humans.

If you're a shift worker and must sleep in the daytime, take your melatonin an hour or two before you plan to sleep and be sure your bedroom is completely dark. An eye mask will help.

For Jet Lag

If you're taking melatonin to address jet lag, take 1–10 mg at bedtime at your destination until you no longer feel the effects of jet lag.

For Viral infections

Dosages up to 20 mg daily may be helpful if you are experiencing any type of immune challenge, especially a virus. At least one study recommends very high dosages —up to 4 mg per pound of body weight per day for people with deadly viral infections. These levels of melatonin should be monitored by a health care practitioner familiar with such usage.

For Cancer

If you are using melatonin to address cancer, please take up to 20 mg daily, especially if you are undergoing chemotherapy. If you are wondering about that high dosage, please re-read Chapter 5 about the many ways melatonin attacks cancer. This dosage is definitely warranted in hormonally-related cancers, like prostate and breast cancer, which can both be very aggressive.

As always, consult your health care professionals for expert guidance. If they have not heard of melatonin use for reasons other than sleep assistance, please copy Chapter 9 and implore them to read it.

WHAT YOU NEED TO KNOW

Melatonin supplements can give you all of the benefits described in this book whether or not you need them as a sleep aid.

You'll benefit from a sustained release supplement taken in the evening, whatever your reason for taking it.

☑ 10 mg of melatonin: Perfect for immune strengthening, restorative sleep and mental well-being.

☑ 20 mg of melatonin: Ideal for protection against viral challenges, tumor risk, rebuilding immune defenses, restoring circadian rhythms and for sleep/wake cycle due to disruptive schedules and travel.

☑ More melatonin may be needed if you have cancer or other serious health issues. Beyond 20 mg daily, please consult a health care provider who has experience with supplements and the various health conditions for which you might use them.

☑ No serious side effects have been associated with melatonin use.

CHAPTER 9

For the Docs: How Melatonin Can Help Your Patients

Dear Health Care Professional,

My name is Jacob Teitelbaum, M.D., a board-certified internal medicine specialist and an integrative physician. I've teamed with Terry Lemerond, a highly-respected supplement researcher and natural health educator for more than 50 years, for this section of this book on melatonin to offer my medical perspective and help underscore the impressive value melatonin can offer your patients.

Melatonin's benefits go far beyond helping sleep. That's why we've encouraged your patient to copy this synopsis and hand it to you, something that is usually anathema in the world of copyrighted books.

In a nutshell, here's what you need to know

Melatonin, a hormone made by the pineal gland, is most often known as a sleep aid. While it is quite effective in overcoming insomnia[1], the research has shown that it offers numerous other health benefits for disease prevention and treatment.

Like other hormones, melatonin is a chemical messenger with well-researched, widespread effects throughout the body. Melatonin also acts as a mitochondrial antioxidant[2] with anti-inflammatory properties.[3]

To give an idea of its power, a review in the medical literature describes it well. "Melatonin, an endigenous indoleamine, is considered an important multitasking molecule with fundamental clinical applications. It is involved in mood modulation, sexual behavior, vasomotor control, and immunomodulation, and influences energy metabolism; moreover, it acts as an oncostatic and anti-aging molecule."[3]

Let's take a look at some of melatonin's actions:

Anti-Aging: We know that balanced circadian rhythms have a profound effect on the entire body. That, plus melatonin's antioxidant, anti-inflammatory, immuno-enhancement, and numerous other properties suggest that it may be a very effective anti-aging molecule.[3,4]

Immune system enhancement: This is probably melatonin's most important role in today's world. It is suggested to be effective against numerous viruses, including COVID-19.[5]

Properties include:

❖ Shows activity against numerous viral challenges including SARS, MERS, avian flu and more

❖ Enhances effectiveness of Natural Killer and T-cells

❖ Increase immune system ability to overcome viral, bacterial, microbial and parasitic infections

❖ Minimal side effects

Cardiovascular health: Antioxidant and anti-inflammatory properties make melatonin a powerful ally against a variety of cardiovascular diseases. Studies show that melatonin:

❖ Reduces cholesterol and triglycerides[6]

❖ Trends towards raising HDL cholesterol[6]

❖ Helps control hypertension,[7] being more effective than salt restriction

❖ Reduces blood coagulation[8]

❖ May be beneficial in congestive heart failure[9]

Cancer prevention: Melatonin's anticancer properties are at least as impressive as its heart supporting ones.[10] It is well researched to:

❖ Induce apoptosis

❖ Inhibit angiogenesis

❖ Inhibit metastasis

❖ Reverse epigenetic damage

❖ Enhance the effectiveness of chemotherapy

❖ Inhibit tumorigenesis through the action of T cells

Melatonin has been shown to be particularly effective in preventing hormonally-related cancers, including breast and prostate cancer. It may also help protect bone marrow cells from the destructive effects of chemo.

Researchers from Baylor University also found that melatonin overcomes cancer patients' almost inevitable resistance to 5-fluorouracil, the chemotherapy drug often used to treat colorectal and other cancers. It may also increase chemotherapy's overall effectiveness.[11]

Sexual health: The anti-inflammatory and anti-oxidative stress effects of melatonin have been shown to:

❖ Result in an increase in successful IVF pregnancies in patients with unexplained infertility[12]

❖ Reverse erectile dysfunction[13]

❖ Increases the probability of success of in vitro fertilization treatments[12]

❖ Levels are also directly associated with sperm motility[14]

❖ Increases the chance of survival for IVF embryos when both men and women are undergoing hormonal enhancement treatment

Control type 2 diabetes: Melatonin may be a helpful tool against type 2 diabetes, although the research on the area is still divided. It has been shown to improve fasting blood sugars.[15]

Sleep disorders, of course: Melatonin is best known for its value as a sleep aid.[1] It restores circadian rhythms and is validated for:

❖ Insomnia

❖ Interrupted sleep

❖ Jet lag

❖ Non-24 sleep/wake disorder

❖ Insomnia as a side effect for various pharmaceuticals, including anti-hypertensives

❖ Insomnia experienced by children on the autism spectrum

Some other conditions (although not limited to these):

❖ Treating and slowing progress of macular degeneration[16] and glaucoma[17]

❖ Relieving chronic pain in sufferers of chronic fatigue syndrome and fibromyalgia, resulting in improved quality of life because of better sleep.[18]

❖ Relief from irritable bowel syndrome[19] and inflammatory bowel disease[20]

❖ Migraine prophylaxis[21]

❖ Markedly decreasing nighttime acid reflux[22]

As you can see, melatonin has broad and valuable effects in improving human health. It is the subject of nearly 27,000 studies published in the National Library of Medicine database.

Since melatonin has a half-life of approximately 60 minutes and a maximum effectiveness range of five hours, an extended-release form of melatonin is preferable in most cases, although immediate release works better for nighttime acid reflux.

As a nutritional supplement researcher for more than 40 years, I personally take melatonin each night and recommend it for most of the people I treat. Given its multiple benefits with minimal risk and low cost, it has a highly favorable risk-benefit assessment. I encourage you to consider it in those that you treat. I am confident your patients will thank you for it.

Jacob Teitelbaum, M.D.
Author of 10 books, including *Real Cause, Real Cure,*
and *From Fatigued to Fantastic!*
AND

Terry Lemerond
Author of *Melatonin: The Miracle for Life*

References

1. *PLoS One.* 2013; 8(5): e63773. Published online 2013 May 17. doi: 10.1371/journal.pone.0063773. Meta-Analysis: Melatonin for the Treatment of Primary Sleep Disorders.

2. *Cell Mol Life Sci.* 2017 Nov;74(21):3863-3881. doi: 10.1007/s00018-017-2609-7. Epub 2017 Sep 1. Melatonin as a mitochondria-targeted antioxidant: one of evolution's best ideas.

3. *Int J Endocrinol.* 2017; 2017: 1835195. doi: 10.1155/2017/1835195. Melatonin as an Anti-Inflammatory Agent Modulating Inflammasome Activation.

4. *Int J Mol Sci.* 2014 Sep; 15(9): 16848–16884. doi: 10.3390/ijms150916848. Melatonin Regulates Aging and Neurodegeneration Through Energy Metabolism, Epigenetics, Autophagy and Circadian Rhythm Pathways.

5. *Virus Res.* 2020 Oct 2; 287: 198108.Doi: 10.1016/j.virusres.2020.198108. Melatonin potentials against viral infections including COVID-19: Current evidence and new findings.

6. *Clin Nutr.* 2018 Dec;37(6 Pt A):1943-1954. doi: 10.1016/j.clnu.2017.11.003. Epub 2017 Nov 16. Effects of melatonin supplementation on blood lipid concentrations: A systematic review and meta-analysis of randomized controlled trials.

7. *Horm Metab Res.* 2019 Mar;51(3):157-164. doi: 10.1055/a-0841-6638. Effects of Melatonin Supplementation On Blood Pressure: A Systematic Review and Meta-Analysis of Randomized Controlled Trials.

8. *J Pineal Res.* 2008 Mar;44(2):127-33. doi: 10.1111/j.1600-079X.2007.00499.x. Oral melatonin reduces blood coagulation activity: a placebo-controlled study in healthy young men.

9. *Molecules.* 2018 Jul; 23(7): 1819.doi: 10.3390/molecules23071819. Melatonin in Heart Failure: A Promising Therapeutic Strategy?

10. *Int J Mol Sci.* 2017 Apr; 18(4): 843. doi: 10.3390/ijms18040843. Melatonin, a Full Service Anti-Cancer Agent: Inhibition of Initiation, Progression and Metastasis

11. *J Pineal Res.* 2017 Mar;62(2). doi: 10.1111/jpi.12380. Melatonin synergizes the chemotherapeutic effect of 5-fluorouracil in colon cancer by suppressing P13K/AKT and NF-kB/iNOS signaling pathways.

12. *Antioxidants* (Basel). 2019 Aug 23;8(9):338. doi: 10.3390/antiox8090338. Impact of Melatonin Supplementation in Women with Unexplained Infertility Undergoing Fertility Treatment.

13. *Int Braz J Urol.* 2018 Jul-Aug; 44(4): 794–799.doi: 10.1590/S1677-5538. IBJU.2017.0663. Low serum melatonin levels are associated with erectile dysfunction.

14. *Cryobiology.* 2020 Aug;95:1-8. doi: 10.1016/j.cryobiol.2020.01.018. Protective effects of melatonin on male fertility preservation and reproductive system.

15. *Horm Metab Res.* 2018 Nov;50(11):783-790. doi: 10.1055/a-0752-8462. The Effects of Melatonin Supplementation on Glycemic Control: A Systematic Review and Meta-Analysis of Randomized Controlled Trials.

16. *Oxid Med Cell Longev.* 2016; 2016: 6819736.doi: 10.1155/2016/6819736. Melatonin in Retinal Physiology and Pathology: The Case of Age-Related Macular Degeneration.

17. *Prog Retin Eye Res.* 2020 Mar;75:100798. doi: 10.1016/j.preteyeres.2019 .100798. Melatonin and the control of intraocular pressure.

18. *Curr Pain Headache Rep.* 2007 Oct;11(5):339-42. doi: 10.1007/s11916-007-0215-3. Melatonin therapy in fibromyalgia.

19. *Gut.* 2005 Oct; 54(10): 1402–1407.doi: 10.1136/gut.2004.062034. Melatonin improves abdominal pain in irritable bowel syndrome patients who have sleep disturbances: a randomised, double blind, placebo controlled study.

20. *Curr Pharm Des.* 2011 Dec;17(38):4372-8. doi: 10.2174/138161211798 999357. Melatonin, a promising supplement in inflammatory bowel disease: a comprehensive review of evidences.

21. *Medicine* (Baltimore). 2019 Jan; 98(3): e14099.doi: 10.1097/MD .0000000000014099. Therapeutic role of melatonin in migraine prophylaxis.A systematic review.

22. *BMC Gastroenterol.* 2010; 10: 7.doi: 10.1186/1471-230X-10-7. The potential therapeutic effect of melatonin in gastro-esophageal reflux disease.

References/Resources

CHAPTER 2: TODAY'S IMPORTANT MELATONIN MESSAGE

Bannerjee, A, Czinn SJ et al. Crosstalk between endoplasmic reticulum stress and anti-viral activities: A novel therapeutic target for COVID-19. *Life Sci.* 2020 Aug 15; 255: 117842.

Silvestri M, Rossi GA, Melatonin: Its possible role in the management of viral infections-a brief review. *Ital J Pediatr.* 2013; 39: 61.

Srinivasan, V., Maestroni, G., Cardinali, D. et al. Melatonin, immune function and aging. *Immun Ageing 2*, 17 (2005). https://doi.org/10.1186/1742-4933-2-17

Sanchez-Barcelo, EJ, Mediavilla Md et al. Clinical Uses of Melatonin: Evaluation in Human Trials. *Current Medicinal Chemistry*, 2020, 17, 2070–95.

CHAPTER 3: MELATONIN FOR LONG LIFE

Reiter RR, Tan DX, Rosales-Corral S et al. Mitochondria: Central Organelles for Melatonin's Antioxidant and Anti-Aging Actions *Molecules*. 2018 Feb; 23(2): 509.

CHAPTER 4: MELATONIN AND A HEALTHY HEART

Koziroq M, Poliwczak AR Duchjnowicz et al. Melatonin treatment improves blood pressure, lipid profile, and parameters of oxidative stress in patients with metabolic syndrome. *J Pineal Res* 2011 Apr;50(3):261–66.

Katsi V, Karagiorgi I, Makris, T et al. The role of melatonin in hypertension. *Cardiovascular Endocrinology*: March 2012 1:1:13-8.

Mohammed-Sartang M, Ghorbani M, Mazloom Z. Effects of melatonin supplementation on blood lipid concentrations: A systematic review and meta-analysis of randomized controlled trials. *Clin Nutr* 2018 Dec;37(6 Pt A):1943–54.

CHAPTER 5: MELATONIN AGAINST CANCER

Miller SC, Pandi, PSR et al. The role of melatonin in immuno-enhancement: potential application in cancer. *Int J Exp Pathol.* 2006 Apr; 87(2): 81–87.

Sanchez-Hidalgo M, Guerrero JM, Vilklegas I et al. Melatonin, a natural programmed cell death inducer in cancer. *Curr Med Chem.* 2012;19(22):3805-21.

Lissoni P, Banri S, Mandala M et. al. Decreased toxicity and increased efficacy of cancer chemotherapy using the pineal hormone melatonin in metastatic solid tumour patients with poor clinical status. *Eur J Cancer.* 1999 Nov;35(12):1688–92.

Gonzalez AG, Rueda N, Alonso-Gonzalez C et. al. Usefulness of melatonin as complementary to chemotherapeutic agents at different stages of the angiogenic process. *Int J Mol Sci.* 2017 Apr; 18(4): 843.

Reiter RJ, Rosales-Corral SA, Tan DX et al. Melatonin, a Full Service Anti-Cancer Agent: Inhibition of Initiation, Progression and Metastasis. *Philos Trans R Soc Lond B Biol Sci.* 2015 May 5;370(1667):20140121.

Samanta S. Melatonin: an endogenous miraculous indolamine, fights against cancer progression. *J Cancer Res Clin Oncol.* 2020 Aug;146(8):1893-1922.

Elmahallawy EK, Mohamed Y, Abdo W et l. Melatonin and Mesenchymal Stem Cells as a Key for Functional Integrity for Liver Cancer Treatment. *Cancer Res Clin Oncol.* 2020 Aug;146(8):1893–1922.

CHAPTER 6: MELATONIN FOR SEXUAL HEALTH

Espina J, Macedo M, Lozano G et al. Impact of Melatonin Supplementation in Women with Unexplained Infertility Undergoing Fertility Treatment. *Antioxidants (Basel).* 2019 Sep; 8(9): 338.

Fernando S, Rombauts L. Melatonin: shedding light on infertility? A review of the recent literature. *J Ovarian Res.* 2014; 7: 98.

Shazia J, Auguste E, Hussain M et al. Sleep and Premenstrual Syndrome. *J Sleep Med Disord.* 2016; 3(5): 1061.

Awad H, Halawa F, Mostafa T et al. Melatonin hormone profile in infertile males. *Int J Androl.* 2006 Jun;29(3):409-13.

Bozkurt A, Karabakan M, Aktas BK et al. Low serum melatonin levels are associated with erectile dysfunction. *Int Braz J Urol.* 2018 Jul–Aug; 44(4): 794–799.

CHAPTER 7: AND FOR SLEEP, OF COURSE

Sketten TL, Magee M, Murray J et al. Efficacy of melatonin with behavioural sleep-wake scheduling for delayed sleep-wake phase disorder: A double-blind, randomised clinical trial. *PLoS Med.* 2018 Jun; 15(6): e1002587.

Gringas P, Nir T, Breddy J et al. Efficacy and Safety of Pediatric Prolonged-Release Melatonin for Insomnia in Children With Autism Spectrum Disorder. *J Am Acad Child Adolesc Psychiatry.* 2017 Nov;56(11):948–957.e4.

Ferracoli-Oda E, Qawasmi A Bloch MH. Meta-analysis: melatonin for the treatment of primary sleep disorders. *PLoS One.* 2013 May 17;8(5):e63773.

CHAPTER 8: KNOW HOW TO MAKE THE RIGHT CHOICE

Tan, D.-X. and Hardeland, R. 2020. Estimated doses of melatonin for treating deadly virus infections: focus on COVID-19. *Melatonin Research.* 3, 3 (Jun. 2020), 276–296.

Index

combined with andrographis,
14, 15
dosages, 58–60
levels in body, 4, 11
production of, 2–3, 9, 20, 26,
31, 39, 41, 51
supplements, 58–60, 65
metabolic syndrome, 27
metastasis, 33, 37–38, 40, 63
migraines, 45, 47, 65
mitochondria, 20, 23, 62

N
naps, 22
nightlights, 54
non 24/7 sleep/wake disorder, 7,
64

O
omeprazole (Prilosec), 45
organelles, 20
ovulation, 41, 42
oxidative stress, 5, 12, 15

P
Pierpaoli, Walter, 2, 3, 17
pineal gland, 2, 3, 26, 31, 39, 41,
51, 61
PMDD. *See* Premenstrual
Dysphoric Disorder (PMDD)
PMS. *See* Premenstrual syndrome
(PMS)
pneumonias, 11, 13, 23
Premenstrual Dysphoric Disorder
(PMDD), 42
Premenstrual syndrome (PMS),
42, 47
Prilosec. *See* omeprazole (Prilosec)

R
Reiter, Russel J., 9–10, 13, 19,
20, 27, 28, 31, 38, 41, 42

S
SARS, 4, 12, 14
selenium, 59, 60
sepsis, 7, 8
sexual health, 5–6, 41–44, 64
shift work, 51, 59
sleep, 1, 7, 8, 22, 28–30, 31, 41,
45, 49–56, 57–58, 61, 64
sleep hygiene, 52–55
sleep-wake cycle. *See* circadian
rhythms
sound, 54
sperm, 44, 64
stress, 4, 50
strokes, 28, 30–31, 52, 56
sunlight, 22, 55

T
television, 9, 53
tinnitus, 46, 47
triglycerides, 27–28, 32, 63

U
ulcers, 45, 47

W
weight, 28, 49, 56
women, 21, 41

Y
yoga, 55

About the Author

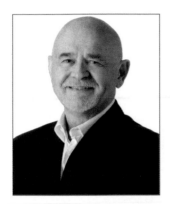

Terry Lemerond is a natural health expert with over 50 years of experience helping people live healthier, happier lives. A much sought-after speaker and accomplished author, Terry shares his wealth of experience and knowledge in health and nutrition through his educational programs, including the *Terry Talks Nutrition* website—TerryTalks Nutrition.com—newsletters, podcasts, webinars, and personal speaking engagements. Terry has also hosted *Terry Talks Nutrition* radio for the past 30 years. His books include *Seven Keys to Vibrant Health, Seven Keys to Unlimited Personal Achievement,* and *50+ Natural Health Secrets Proven to Change Your Life.* Terry continues to author and co-author books to educate everyone on the steps they can take to live a more healthy, vibrant life.

His continual dedication, energy, and zeal are part of his ongoing mission—to help us all improve our health.